Table Of Contents

Chapter 1: Understanding IBS and the Gut Microbiome

What is IBS?

Irritable Bowel Syndrome, commonly known as IBS, is a chronic gastrointestinal disorder that affects millions of people worldwide. It is a functional disorder, meaning that there is no visible damage to the digestive tract, but rather a disruption in the normal functioning of the bowels. Symptoms of IBS can vary widely from person to person and may include abdominal pain, bloating, diarrhea, constipation, or a combination of both.

IBS is believed to be caused by a variety of factors, including genetics, diet, stress, and an imbalance in the gut microbiome. The gut microbiome refers to the community of bacteria and other microorganisms that reside in the digestive tract and play a crucial role in digestion, nutrient absorption, and immune function. When this delicate balance is disrupted, it can lead to inflammation and dysfunction in the gut, contributing to the development of IBS.

Many individuals with IBS turn to natural remedies to help manage their symptoms and improve their overall gut health. These remedies may include dietary changes, such as increasing fiber intake, eliminating trigger foods, and incorporating probiotic-rich foods into the diet. Herbal supplements, such as peppermint oil and aloe vera, have also been shown to have a beneficial effect on IBS symptoms.

In addition to dietary and herbal remedies, lifestyle changes can also play a significant role in managing IBS. Stress management techniques, such as meditation, yoga, and deep breathing exercises, can help reduce the frequency and severity of IBS symptoms. Regular exercise, adequate sleep, and staying hydrated are also important factors in maintaining gut health and managing IBS.

Overall, understanding the underlying causes of IBS, such as gut microbiome imbalances, and incorporating natural remedies into your daily routine can help alleviate symptoms, improve gut health, and enhance overall well-being. By nourishing your gut and healing your body through natural means, you can take control of your IBS and live a healthier, happier life.

The Role of the Gut Microbiome in IBS

The gut microbiome plays a crucial role in the development and management of Irritable Bowel Syndrome (IBS). The gut microbiome refers to the trillions of bacteria, fungi, and other microorganisms that live in our digestive tract. These microorganisms help break down food, produce essential nutrients, and even regulate our immune system. In individuals with IBS, the balance of these microorganisms is disrupted, leading to symptoms such as bloating, gas, diarrhea, and constipation.

Research has shown that individuals with IBS have a different composition of gut bacteria compared to healthy individuals. This imbalance, known as dysbiosis, can contribute to inflammation and increased gut permeability, both of which are associated with IBS symptoms. By nourishing and supporting a healthy gut microbiome, individuals with IBS can potentially reduce their symptoms and improve their overall gut health.

Natural remedies such as probiotics, prebiotics, and dietary changes can help restore balance to the gut microbiome and alleviate symptoms of IBS. Probiotics are beneficial bacteria that can help replenish the gut microbiome and improve digestion. Prebiotics, on the other hand, are indigestible fibers that feed the good bacteria in the gut, promoting their growth and diversity. By incorporating these natural remedies into their daily routine, individuals with IBS can support their gut health and potentially reduce their symptoms.

In addition to probiotics and prebiotics, dietary changes can also play a significant role in improving gut health and managing IBS symptoms. Certain foods, such as high-FODMAP foods, gluten, and dairy, can trigger symptoms in individuals with IBS. By identifying and eliminating these trigger foods from their diet, individuals with IBS can reduce inflammation in the gut and improve their overall gut health. Incorporating more fiber-rich foods, such as fruits, vegetables, and whole grains, can also help support a healthy gut microbiome and improve digestion.

Overall, understanding the role of the gut microbiome in IBS is essential for individuals looking to manage their symptoms and improve their gut health. By incorporating natural remedies such as probiotics, prebiotics, and dietary changes into their daily routine, individuals with IBS can support a healthy gut microbiome and potentially reduce their symptoms. Nourishing the gut microbiome is a key component of managing IBS and promoting overall gut health.

How Gut Health Impacts Overall Well-being

In recent years, the importance of gut health has gained significant attention in the medical and wellness communities. Research has shown that the health of our gut microbiome plays a crucial role in our overall well-being, including our immune function, mental health, and even our weight management. For individuals suffering from irritable bowel syndrome (IBS), maintaining a healthy gut is particularly important, as imbalances in the gut microbiome can exacerbate symptoms and contribute to digestive issues.

The gut microbiome is a complex ecosystem of trillions of bacteria, viruses, and fungi that reside in our digestive tract. These microorganisms play a vital role in digestion, nutrient absorption, and immune function. When the balance of these microbes is disrupted, it can lead to inflammation, digestive issues, and other health problems. For individuals with IBS, an imbalance in the gut microbiome can trigger symptoms such as abdominal pain, bloating, diarrhea, and constipation.

Fortunately, there are natural remedies that can help nourish the gut and promote a healthy balance of gut bacteria. Probiotics, which are beneficial bacteria that can help restore balance to the gut microbiome, are commonly used to support digestive health in individuals with IBS. Prebiotics, which are non-digestible fibers that feed the good bacteria in the gut, can also promote a healthy gut microbiome and improve digestive function.

In addition to probiotics and prebiotics, dietary changes can also play a significant role in improving gut health and managing symptoms of IBS. Eating a diet rich in fiber, fruits, vegetables, and whole grains can help support a healthy gut microbiome and reduce inflammation in the digestive tract. Avoiding trigger foods such as dairy, gluten, and high-fat foods can also help alleviate symptoms and promote gut health.

By taking steps to nourish the gut and support a healthy balance of gut bacteria, individuals with IBS can improve their overall well-being and reduce symptoms. Incorporating natural remedies such as probiotics, prebiotics, and dietary changes can help restore balance to the gut microbiome and promote digestive health. With a focus on gut health, individuals with IBS can take control of their symptoms and improve their quality of life.

Chapter 2: Common Symptoms and Triggers of IBS

Identifying Common Symptoms of IBS

Irritable Bowel Syndrome (IBS) is a common digestive disorder that affects many individuals over the age of 18. It is important to be able to recognize the common symptoms of IBS in order to seek proper treatment and management. One of the key symptoms of IBS is abdominal pain or discomfort that is often relieved by a bowel movement. This pain may be crampy in nature and can vary in intensity from mild to severe.

Another common symptom of IBS is changes in bowel habits. This can include diarrhea, constipation, or a combination of both. Individuals with IBS may experience frequent and urgent bowel movements, or may have difficulty passing stools. It is important to pay attention to these changes in order to accurately diagnose and treat IBS.

Bloating and gas are also common symptoms of IBS. Individuals with IBS may experience excess gas production, leading to bloating and discomfort. This can be exacerbated by certain foods or stress. It is important to identify triggers that may worsen these symptoms in order to manage IBS effectively.

In addition to physical symptoms, individuals with IBS may also experience emotional symptoms such as anxiety or depression. The gut-brain connection is strong, and stress can often trigger or exacerbate IBS symptoms. It is important to address both physical and emotional symptoms in order to effectively manage IBS.

Overall, recognizing the common symptoms of IBS is crucial in order to seek proper treatment and management. By identifying and addressing these symptoms, individuals can take control of their health and improve their quality of life. Natural remedies, such as dietary changes and stress management techniques, can be effective in managing IBS symptoms and promoting gut health.

Understanding Triggers for IBS Flare-ups

Living with Irritable Bowel Syndrome (IBS) can be challenging, especially when flare-ups occur unexpectedly. It is important for individuals with IBS to identify their triggers in order to better manage their symptoms and improve their overall quality of life. By understanding what can cause flare-ups, individuals can take proactive steps to prevent them and minimize their impact on their daily routine.

One of the most common triggers for IBS flare-ups is certain foods. Foods high in FODMAPs, such as garlic, onions, and certain dairy products, can exacerbate symptoms in individuals with IBS. Additionally, spicy foods, caffeine, and alcohol are known to trigger flare-ups in some people. By keeping a food diary and paying attention to how different foods affect their symptoms, individuals with IBS can identify their specific triggers and make informed decisions about their diet.

Stress and anxiety are also common triggers for IBS flare-ups. The gut-brain connection is well-documented, and emotional stress can have a direct impact on gut health. Mind-body practices such as yoga, meditation, and deep breathing exercises can help individuals with IBS manage their stress levels and reduce the likelihood of flare-ups. It is important for individuals with IBS to prioritize their mental health and find healthy coping mechanisms for stress.

Another common trigger for IBS flare-ups is poor sleep quality. Lack of sleep can disrupt the gut microbiome and lead to increased inflammation in the digestive tract. Establishing a regular sleep routine, practicing good sleep hygiene, and creating a calming bedtime routine can help individuals with IBS improve their sleep quality and reduce the risk of flare-ups. Prioritizing rest and relaxation is essential for managing IBS symptoms and promoting overall gut health.

In addition to food, stress, and sleep, other triggers for IBS flare-ups may include hormonal fluctuations, medications, and environmental factors. By working with a healthcare provider or nutritionist, individuals with IBS can create a personalized plan to identify and address their triggers. By taking a holistic approach to managing IBS, individuals can nourish their gut, heal their body, and live a more vibrant and fulfilling life.

The Connection Between Stress and IBS

Stress is a common trigger for many individuals suffering from Irritable Bowel Syndrome (IBS). The connection between stress and IBS is complex, as stress can exacerbate symptoms of IBS and vice versa. Research has shown that stress can lead to changes in the gut microbiome, which plays a crucial role in the development and management of IBS. When stress levels are high, the gut microbiome can become imbalanced, leading to increased inflammation and digestive issues.

One of the key ways in which stress affects IBS is through the gut-brain axis, a bidirectional communication system between the brain and the gut. When we experience stress, the brain sends signals to the gut, triggering symptoms such as cramping, bloating, and diarrhea. This can lead to a vicious cycle where stress exacerbates IBS symptoms, causing further stress and worsening of symptoms.

Natural remedies can play a crucial role in managing both stress and IBS symptoms. By addressing the root cause of stress and supporting the gut microbiome, natural remedies can help alleviate symptoms and improve overall gut health. Some natural remedies that have been shown to be effective in managing stress and IBS include probiotics, herbal supplements, and mind-body techniques such as meditation and yoga.

Probiotics are beneficial bacteria that can help restore balance to the gut microbiome and reduce inflammation in the gut. Studies have shown that probiotics can improve symptoms of IBS, such as bloating, gas, and diarrhea. Herbal supplements such as peppermint oil and ginger can also help relieve symptoms of IBS and reduce stress. These natural remedies can be a safe and effective alternative to traditional medications for managing IBS.

In conclusion, the connection between stress and IBS is a complex and multifaceted one. By addressing both stress and gut health through natural remedies, individuals with IBS can find relief from their symptoms and improve their overall quality of life. It is important for those suffering from IBS to work with a healthcare provider to develop a comprehensive treatment plan that includes natural remedies tailored to their individual needs.

Chapter 3: Natural Remedies for Managing IBS Symptoms

Dietary Changes for IBS Relief

One of the most effective ways to manage the symptoms of Irritable Bowel Syndrome (IBS) is through dietary changes. By making small adjustments to your diet, you can alleviate discomfort and reduce the frequency of flare-ups. It is important to note that everyone's body is different, so what works for one person may not work for another. However, there are some general guidelines that can help you find relief from IBS symptoms.

First and foremost, it is essential to identify trigger foods that may exacerbate your symptoms. Common trigger foods for individuals with IBS include dairy products, gluten, and high-fat foods. Keeping a food diary can help you track your symptoms and identify any patterns that may be linked to specific foods. Once you have identified trigger foods, try to eliminate them from your diet and see if your symptoms improve.

In addition to avoiding trigger foods, it is important to focus on incorporating gut-friendly foods into your diet. Foods high in fiber, such as fruits, vegetables, and whole grains, can help regulate digestion and alleviate symptoms of IBS. Probiotic-rich foods, such as yogurt, kefir, and sauerkraut, can also help promote a healthy gut microbiome and reduce inflammation in the digestive tract. By incorporating these foods into your diet, you can support your gut health and reduce symptoms of IBS.

Another important dietary change for IBS relief is to eat smaller, more frequent meals throughout the day. Large meals can put added stress on the digestive system and exacerbate symptoms of bloating, gas, and abdominal pain. By eating smaller meals more frequently, you can help regulate digestion and reduce discomfort. Additionally, it is important to stay hydrated by drinking plenty of water throughout the day, as dehydration can worsen symptoms of IBS.

Overall, making dietary changes for IBS relief is a process of trial and error. It may take time to identify trigger foods and find a diet that works best for your body. However, by focusing on gut-friendly foods, avoiding trigger foods, and eating smaller, more frequent meals, you can support your gut health and reduce symptoms of IBS naturally. Remember to consult with a healthcare provider or nutritionist before making significant changes to your diet, especially if you have underlying health conditions.

Herbal Supplements for Gut Health

When it comes to managing irritable bowel syndrome (IBS) and promoting a healthy gut microbiome, herbal supplements can be a powerful ally. These natural remedies have been used for centuries to support digestive health and alleviate symptoms such as bloating, gas, and abdominal pain. By incorporating herbal supplements into your daily routine, you can nourish your gut and heal your body from the inside out.

One of the most popular herbal supplements for gut health is peppermint oil. Peppermint oil has been shown to relax the muscles of the digestive tract, which can help to alleviate symptoms of IBS such as cramping and bloating. Additionally, peppermint oil has anti-inflammatory properties that can help to reduce inflammation in the gut, making it a great choice for those with IBS.

Another herbal supplement that is beneficial for gut health is ginger. Ginger has long been used to aid digestion and soothe an upset stomach. It has anti-inflammatory properties that can help to reduce inflammation in the gut, as well as anti-nausea properties that can help to alleviate symptoms of IBS such as nausea and vomiting. Ginger can be taken in supplement form or added to food and beverages for an extra boost of gut-healing goodness.

Turmeric is another herbal supplement that can support gut health. Turmeric contains curcumin, a compound that has powerful anti-inflammatory and antioxidant properties. By reducing inflammation in the gut, turmeric can help to alleviate symptoms of IBS such as abdominal pain and discomfort. Turmeric can be taken in supplement form or added to curries, soups, and smoothies for a delicious and healing boost.

In addition to peppermint oil, ginger, and turmeric, there are many other herbal supplements that can support gut health and alleviate symptoms of IBS. Some other popular options include marshmallow root, slippery elm, and chamomile. These herbs can help to soothe inflammation in the gut, improve digestion, and promote overall gut health. When choosing herbal supplements for gut health, it's important to consult with a healthcare provider or naturopath to ensure that you are selecting the right supplements for your individual needs and health goals. By incorporating herbal supplements into your daily routine, you can nourish your gut, heal your body, and take control of your IBS symptoms naturally.

Probiotics and Prebiotics for Balancing Gut Flora

Probiotics and prebiotics play a crucial role in balancing the gut flora, which is essential for maintaining good digestive health. In individuals with irritable bowel syndrome (IBS), the delicate balance of bacteria in the gut is often disrupted, leading to symptoms such as bloating, gas, diarrhea, and constipation. By incorporating probiotics and prebiotics into your diet, you can help restore this balance and alleviate some of the discomfort associated with IBS.

Probiotics are live bacteria and yeasts that are beneficial for your digestive system. They help to restore the natural balance of bacteria in the gut and promote overall gut health. Some studies have shown that certain strains of probiotics can help reduce symptoms of IBS, such as abdominal pain and bloating. Probiotics are commonly found in fermented foods like yogurt, kefir, sauerkraut, and kimchi, as well as in supplement form. When choosing a probiotic supplement, look for one that contains a variety of strains and a high number of colony-forming units (CFUs) to ensure effectiveness.

Prebiotics, on the other hand, are non-digestible fibers that serve as food for the beneficial bacteria in the gut. By consuming prebiotic-rich foods like bananas, onions, garlic, and asparagus, you can help nourish the good bacteria in your gut and promote their growth. Prebiotics can also help improve the overall balance of bacteria in the gut and support digestive health. Including a variety of prebiotic foods in your diet can help enhance the effectiveness of probiotics and further support gut health.

Combining probiotics and prebiotics in your diet can have a synergistic effect on gut health, as they work together to promote the growth of beneficial bacteria and maintain a healthy balance of gut flora. This can help alleviate symptoms of IBS and improve overall digestive function. It's important to note that everyone's gut microbiome is unique, so it may take some trial and error to find the right combination of probiotics and prebiotics that work best for you. Consulting with a healthcare provider or a registered dietitian can help you develop a personalized plan for incorporating probiotics and prebiotics into your diet to support gut health and manage symptoms of IBS.

Incorporating probiotics and prebiotics into your daily routine can be a simple and effective way to support your gut health naturally. By nourishing your gut with beneficial bacteria and the right nutrients, you can help restore balance to your gut flora and improve digestive function. Taking steps to promote a healthy gut microbiome through diet and lifestyle changes can be an important aspect of managing IBS symptoms and achieving overall wellness.

Chapter 4: Lifestyle Changes for Long-term Relief

Stress Management Techniques for IBS

Living with irritable bowel syndrome (IBS) can be incredibly challenging, as the symptoms can often be triggered or exacerbated by stress. In order to effectively manage IBS, it is crucial to incorporate stress management techniques into your daily routine. By addressing stress and anxiety, you can help alleviate the symptoms of IBS and improve your overall quality of life.

One of the most effective stress management techniques for IBS is mindfulness meditation. By practicing mindfulness, you can learn to focus on the present moment and cultivate a sense of calm and relaxation. This can help reduce the impact of stress on your gut, leading to fewer IBS flare-ups and a reduction in symptoms such as bloating, gas, and abdominal pain.

Another helpful technique for managing stress with IBS is deep breathing exercises. By taking slow, deep breaths, you can activate your body's relaxation response and help calm your nervous system. Deep breathing can be done anywhere, at any time, making it a convenient tool for managing stress on the go.

Regular exercise is another important component of stress management for IBS. Physical activity has been shown to reduce stress levels, improve mood, and promote overall well-being. By incorporating regular exercise into your routine, you can help alleviate the symptoms of IBS and reduce the impact of stress on your gut.

In addition to these techniques, it is also important to prioritize self-care and relaxation. This may include activities such as reading, listening to music, taking a warm bath, or spending time in nature. By making time for self-care, you can help reduce stress levels and improve your overall mental and physical health, leading to better management of IBS symptoms. By incorporating these stress management techniques into your daily routine, you can help alleviate the symptoms of IBS and improve your overall quality of life.

Exercise and Physical Activity for Gut Health

Exercise and physical activity play a crucial role in maintaining gut health, especially for those suffering from Irritable Bowel Syndrome (IBS). Regular exercise has been shown to improve digestion, reduce inflammation, and promote the growth of beneficial bacteria in the gut. Physical activity can also help relieve symptoms of IBS such as bloating, gas, and abdominal pain. By incorporating exercise into your daily routine, you can support your gut health and overall well-being.

One of the key benefits of exercise for gut health is its ability to reduce inflammation in the body. Chronic inflammation in the gut is a common factor in many digestive disorders, including IBS. By engaging in regular physical activity, you can help lower levels of inflammation in your gut, leading to improved digestion and reduced symptoms of IBS. Exercise also helps regulate the immune system, which plays a crucial role in maintaining a healthy gut microbiome.

In addition to reducing inflammation, exercise can also promote the growth of beneficial bacteria in the gut. These friendly microbes play a crucial role in digestion, nutrient absorption, and overall gut health. By staying active, you can help create a more favorable environment for these good bacteria to thrive, leading to a healthier gut microbiome. This can result in improved digestion, reduced bloating, and better overall gut function for those with IBS.

Physical activity can also help alleviate common symptoms of IBS, such as bloating, gas, and abdominal pain. Exercise helps stimulate the muscles in the digestive tract, promoting more regular bowel movements and reducing discomfort. By incorporating activities such as walking, yoga, or strength training into your routine, you can help support healthy digestion and relieve symptoms of IBS. Additionally, exercise can help manage stress, which is a common trigger for IBS flare-ups.

Overall, incorporating exercise and physical activity into your daily routine can have a positive impact on your gut health and overall well-being, especially for those suffering from IBS. By reducing inflammation, promoting the growth of beneficial bacteria, and alleviating common symptoms of IBS, exercise can be a powerful natural remedy for improving gut health. Whether you prefer gentle activities like yoga or more intense workouts like running, finding ways to stay active can help nourish your gut and heal your body from the inside out.

Importance of Adequate Sleep for Managing IBS

In the world of managing irritable bowel syndrome (IBS), it is crucial to recognize the importance of adequate sleep in maintaining gut health. Sleep plays a significant role in regulating our body's natural processes, including digestion and gut function. For individuals struggling with IBS, getting enough quality sleep can make a world of difference in managing symptoms and improving overall well-being.

Research has shown that inadequate sleep can have a direct impact on gut health, leading to increased inflammation, altered gut microbiome composition, and heightened sensitivity to gastrointestinal symptoms. By prioritizing a consistent sleep schedule and aiming for 7-9 hours of quality rest each night, individuals with IBS can support their gut health and reduce the severity of symptoms.

Furthermore, adequate sleep is essential for supporting the body's immune system and regulating stress levels, both of which play a significant role in IBS management. When we are sleep-deprived, our bodies are more susceptible to inflammation and oxidative stress, which can exacerbate symptoms of IBS. By prioritizing restful sleep, individuals can strengthen their immune system and reduce the impact of stress on gut health, leading to improved overall well-being.

In addition to supporting gut health, adequate sleep can also improve cognitive function, mood, and energy levels - all of which can be negatively impacted by IBS symptoms. By getting enough rest each night, individuals with IBS can better cope with the challenges of their condition and approach their treatment with a clearer mind and more positive outlook.

In conclusion, the importance of adequate sleep for managing IBS cannot be overstated. By prioritizing restful sleep and establishing healthy sleep habits, individuals can support their gut health, reduce inflammation and stress, and improve overall well-being. Incorporating adequate sleep into a comprehensive treatment plan for IBS can lead to significant improvements in symptoms and quality of life.

Chapter 5: Seeking Professional Help for Severe Cases

When to Consult a Doctor for IBS Symptoms

If you are experiencing symptoms of Irritable Bowel Syndrome (IBS), it is important to know when it is time to consult a doctor for help. While many cases of IBS can be managed with lifestyle changes and natural remedies, there are certain situations where professional medical advice is necessary. In this subchapter, we will discuss when it is appropriate to seek help from a healthcare provider for your IBS symptoms.

One of the key indicators that it may be time to consult a doctor for your IBS symptoms is if they are significantly impacting your quality of life. If you are experiencing frequent and severe abdominal pain, bloating, diarrhea, or constipation that is interfering with your daily activities, it is important to seek medical attention. A doctor can help you identify the underlying causes of your symptoms and develop a treatment plan to manage them effectively.

Another reason to consult a doctor for IBS symptoms is if you are experiencing unexplained weight loss or a change in your bowel habits that lasts for more than a few weeks. These can be signs of a more serious underlying condition that may require medical intervention. A doctor can perform tests to rule out other potential causes of your symptoms and provide you with a proper diagnosis and treatment plan.

If you have tried various natural remedies for IBS and have not seen any improvement in your symptoms, it may be time to consult a doctor. While natural remedies can be effective for many people, they are not always a one-size-fits-all solution. A doctor can help you explore other treatment options, such as prescription medications or dietary changes, that may be more effective in managing your symptoms.

Additionally, if you are experiencing symptoms of IBS for the first time or if your symptoms have suddenly worsened, it is important to consult a doctor. These changes in your symptoms could be a sign of a new underlying condition or a flare-up of your IBS that may require medical intervention. A doctor can help you determine the cause of your symptoms and develop a personalized treatment plan to address them.

In conclusion, knowing when to consult a doctor for your IBS symptoms is crucial for managing your condition effectively. If your symptoms are significantly impacting your quality of life, if you are experiencing unexplained weight loss or changes in your bowel habits, if natural remedies have not been effective, or if your symptoms have suddenly worsened, it is important to seek medical attention. A doctor can help you identify the underlying causes of your symptoms and develop a treatment plan that is tailored to your individual needs.

Available Treatments for Severe IBS Cases

For individuals suffering from severe cases of Irritable Bowel Syndrome (IBS), finding effective treatments can be a daunting task. While mild cases of IBS can often be managed with dietary changes and stress-reducing techniques, more severe cases may require additional interventions. In this chapter, we will explore some of the available treatments for severe IBS cases, focusing on natural remedies that nourish the gut and heal the body.

One of the most promising treatments for severe IBS cases is the use of probiotics. Probiotics are live bacteria and yeasts that are good for your digestive system. Studies have shown that probiotics can help to rebalance the gut microbiome, reducing inflammation and improving symptoms of IBS. By introducing beneficial bacteria into the gut, probiotics can help to restore the natural balance of microorganisms, leading to improved digestion and reduced symptoms of IBS.

Another natural remedy that has shown promise in treating severe IBS cases is the use of herbal supplements. Certain herbs, such as peppermint, ginger, and turmeric, have been shown to have anti-inflammatory and soothing effects on the digestive system. These herbs can help to calm the gut, reduce bloating and gas, and alleviate abdominal pain. By incorporating these herbal supplements into your daily routine, you may be able to find relief from the symptoms of severe IBS.

In addition to probiotics and herbal supplements, dietary changes can also play a crucial role in managing severe cases of IBS. Certain foods, such as gluten, dairy, and high-FODMAP foods, can trigger symptoms of IBS in some individuals. By eliminating these trigger foods from your diet and focusing on whole, nutrient-dense foods, you may be able to reduce inflammation in the gut and improve your overall digestive health. Working with a registered dietitian or nutritionist can help you develop a personalized diet plan that meets your nutritional needs while also supporting your gut health.

It is important to remember that finding the right treatment for severe IBS cases may require some trial and error. What works for one individual may not work for another, so it is essential to be patient and persistent in your quest for relief. By exploring natural remedies, such as probiotics, herbal supplements, and dietary changes, you may be able to find a treatment plan that works for you. Remember to consult with your healthcare provider before making any significant changes to your treatment plan, and never hesitate to seek support from a qualified healthcare professional. With dedication and perseverance, you can find relief from the symptoms of severe IBS and nourish your gut for optimal health and well-being.

Working with a Dietitian for Personalized Nutrition Plans

Working with a dietitian can be a game-changer for those looking to manage their IBS symptoms through personalized nutrition plans.

These professionals are trained to help individuals identify trigger foods, create balanced meal plans, and make dietary changes that can significantly improve gut health. By working closely with a dietitian, individuals can gain a better understanding of their unique dietary needs and develop a plan that works best for their bodies.

One of the key benefits of working with a dietitian is the personalized approach they take to crafting nutrition plans. Unlike generic diets or one-size-fits-all meal plans, a dietitian will work with individuals to identify their specific trigger foods and create a plan that is tailored to their needs. This personalized approach can help individuals avoid foods that exacerbate their symptoms and focus on incorporating gut-friendly foods that nourish their bodies.

In addition to creating personalized nutrition plans, dietitians can also provide valuable education and support to individuals looking to manage their IBS symptoms naturally. By educating individuals on the connection between diet and gut health, dietitians can empower them to make informed decisions about their food choices and lifestyle habits. This knowledge can be incredibly empowering and can help individuals take control of their health and well-being.

Working with a dietitian can also help individuals navigate the often overwhelming world of natural remedies for IBS. With so many different diets, supplements, and protocols available, it can be challenging to know where to start. A dietitian can help individuals sift through the information and identify which natural remedies may be most beneficial for their specific symptoms and needs.

Overall, working with a dietitian for personalized nutrition plans can be a transformative experience for individuals looking to manage their IBS symptoms naturally. By taking a personalized approach to nutrition, educating individuals on the connection between diet and gut health, and helping them navigate the world of natural remedies, dietitians can empower individuals to take control of their health and well-being. If you are struggling with IBS symptoms, consider reaching out to a dietitian to see how they can help you on your journey to better gut health.

Chapter 6: Maintaining Gut Health for Overall Wellness

Incorporating Probiotic-Rich Foods into Your Diet

One of the most effective ways to support your gut health and manage symptoms of irritable bowel syndrome (IBS) is by incorporating probiotic-rich foods into your diet. Probiotics are beneficial bacteria that can help restore the balance of your gut microbiome and improve digestion. By including these foods in your daily meals, you can promote a healthy gut environment and reduce the frequency and severity of IBS symptoms.

Yogurt is one of the most well-known probiotic-rich foods and can be easily incorporated into your diet. Look for varieties that contain live and active cultures, as these are the beneficial bacteria that will support your gut health. You can enjoy yogurt on its own, mixed with fruit and nuts, or blended into smoothies for a delicious and nutritious snack or breakfast option.

Another great source of probiotics is fermented foods like kimchi, sauerkraut, and kombucha. These foods are rich in beneficial bacteria that can help improve digestion and reduce inflammation in the gut. Try adding a small serving of fermented vegetables to your meals or sipping on a glass of kombucha as a refreshing beverage option. These foods can be a tasty way to support your gut health and manage IBS symptoms naturally.

In addition to yogurt and fermented foods, you can also incorporate other probiotic-rich options into your diet, such as kefir, miso, and tempeh. These foods contain a variety of beneficial bacteria strains that can help promote a healthy gut microbiome and improve overall digestive function. Experiment with different recipes and meal ideas to find creative ways to include these probiotic-rich foods in your daily meals.

Remember that it's important to consume a variety of probiotic-rich foods to ensure you're getting a diverse range of beneficial bacteria strains. By incorporating these foods into your diet regularly, you can support your gut health, improve digestion, and reduce symptoms of IBS naturally. Talk to your healthcare provider or a registered dietitian for personalized recommendations on how to incorporate probiotic-rich foods into your diet to manage your IBS symptoms effectively.

The Benefits of Regular Exercise for Gut Health

Regular exercise is not only beneficial for maintaining physical fitness and overall health, but it also plays a crucial role in promoting gut health. Studies have shown that engaging in regular physical activity can help improve the balance of bacteria in the gut, known as the gut microbiome. This can lead to a reduction in symptoms of irritable bowel syndrome (IBS) and other gut-related issues.

One of the key benefits of exercise for gut health is its ability to reduce inflammation in the body. Chronic inflammation in the gut is a common factor in the development of IBS and other digestive disorders. By engaging in regular physical activity, individuals can help lower levels of inflammation in the gut, which can lead to a decrease in symptoms such as bloating, gas, and abdominal pain.

In addition to reducing inflammation, exercise can also help improve the motility of the intestines. This means that food and waste move through the digestive system more efficiently, reducing the risk of constipation and promoting regular bowel movements. By incorporating regular exercise into your routine, you can help support healthy digestion and prevent issues such as constipation or diarrhea.

Furthermore, exercise has been shown to have a positive impact on mental health, which is closely linked to gut health. Stress and anxiety can exacerbate symptoms of IBS and other digestive disorders, leading to increased discomfort and pain. Engaging in regular physical activity can help reduce stress levels, improve mood, and promote relaxation, all of which can have a beneficial effect on gut health.

Overall, incorporating regular exercise into your routine can have a profound impact on your gut health and overall well-being. By reducing inflammation, improving motility, and supporting mental health, exercise can help alleviate symptoms of IBS and other digestive issues. Whether you prefer yoga, running, or weightlifting, finding a form of exercise that you enjoy and can commit to regularly can be a valuable tool in managing gut health naturally.

Mindfulness Practices for Gut-Brain Connection

In this subchapter, we will explore mindfulness practices that can help improve the gut-brain connection, a crucial component in managing irritable bowel syndrome (IBS) symptoms. Mindfulness involves being fully present and aware of your thoughts, emotions, and bodily sensations without judgment. By practicing mindfulness, you can reduce stress, anxiety, and other negative emotions that can trigger IBS flare-ups.

One mindfulness practice that can benefit the gut-brain connection is deep breathing exercises. Deep breathing can help calm the nervous system, reduce stress, and promote relaxation. By taking slow, deep breaths, you can signal to your body that it is safe and decrease the fight-or-flight response that can exacerbate IBS symptoms. Practicing deep breathing for just a few minutes each day can have a significant impact on your gut health.

Another mindfulness practice that can support the gut-brain connection is meditation. Meditation involves focusing your attention on the present moment and quieting the mind. By meditating regularly, you can train your brain to respond more calmly to stressors and reduce the negative impact of anxiety on your gut health. Research has shown that meditation can improve

IBS symptoms by reducing inflammation, strengthening the gut barrier, and balancing the gut microbiome.

Yoga is another mindfulness practice that can help improve the gut-brain connection and alleviate IBS symptoms. Yoga combines physical postures, breathing exercises, and meditation to promote relaxation, reduce stress, and improve digestive health. By practicing yoga regularly, you can increase body awareness, regulate your breathing, and reduce muscle tension that can contribute to IBS flare-ups. Yoga has been shown to improve gut motility, reduce bloating, and enhance overall gut function.

Incorporating mindfulness practices into your daily routine can have a positive impact on your gut health and overall well-being. By reducing stress, anxiety, and other negative emotions, you can support the gut-brain connection and improve IBS symptoms. Whether you choose deep breathing exercises, meditation, yoga, or a combination of these practices, mindfulness can be a powerful tool in managing IBS and promoting natural remedies for gut health. Take the time to nurture your gut-brain connection and see the transformative effects on your digestive health.

Chapter 7: Recipes and Meal Plans for IBS Relief

IBS-Friendly Breakfast Ideas

If you suffer from Irritable Bowel Syndrome (IBS), you know how important it is to start your day off right with a healthy and gut-friendly breakfast. In this subchapter, we will explore some delicious and nutritious breakfast ideas that are gentle on the gut and can help alleviate IBS symptoms. By incorporating these IBS-friendly breakfast options into your daily routine, you can nourish your gut and heal your body from the inside out.

One delicious and IBS-friendly breakfast idea is a smoothie made with gut-friendly ingredients such as bananas, strawberries, and almond milk. Bananas are rich in fiber and can help regulate digestion, while strawberries are packed with antioxidants that can reduce inflammation in the gut. Almond milk is a great alternative to dairy for those with lactose intolerance, and it is easy on the digestive system. Simply blend these ingredients together for a refreshing and nutritious breakfast option.

Another great IBS-friendly breakfast idea is overnight oats. Oats are a great source of soluble fiber, which can help regulate bowel movements and ease symptoms of IBS. To make overnight oats, simply combine oats with your choice of milk (such as almond or coconut milk), chia seeds, and a sweetener like honey or maple syrup. Let the mixture sit in the refrigerator overnight, and in the morning, you will have a delicious and gut-friendly breakfast ready to enjoy.

For those who prefer a savory breakfast option, a vegetable omelette is a great choice for those with IBS. Eggs are a good source of protein and can be easily digested, while vegetables like spinach, bell peppers, and mushrooms are rich in vitamins and minerals that can support gut health. You can customize your omelette with your favorite veggies and seasonings for a delicious and satisfying breakfast that won't aggravate your IBS symptoms.

If you are looking for a quick and easy IBS-friendly breakfast option, a bowl of Greek yogurt topped with low-FODMAP fruits like blueberries or kiwi is a great choice. Greek yogurt is rich in probiotics that can help balance the gut microbiome and improve digestion, while low-FODMAP fruits are less likely to cause digestive issues for those with IBS. This simple breakfast option is perfect for those on the go who still want to prioritize their gut health.

In conclusion, starting your day with an IBS-friendly breakfast is essential for managing your symptoms and nourishing your gut. By incorporating these delicious and nutritious breakfast ideas into your daily routine, you can support your gut health and overall well-being. Experiment with these options and find what works best for you and your body to alleviate IBS symptoms and promote a healthy gut microbiome.

Gut-Healing Lunch and Dinner Recipes

In this subchapter, we will explore some delicious and gut-healing lunch and dinner recipes that are perfect for those looking to nourish their gut and heal their body. These recipes are specifically designed to help alleviate symptoms of IBS and promote a healthy gut microbiome. By incorporating these recipes into your meal plan, you can take a proactive approach to managing your IBS symptoms and improving your overall gut health.

One of the key ingredients in these recipes is fiber-rich foods such as fruits, vegetables, and whole grains. Fiber is essential for maintaining a healthy digestive system and promoting good gut bacteria. By including plenty of fiber in your diet, you can help to regulate your bowel movements and reduce symptoms of IBS like bloating and constipation. Some great sources of fiber to include in your meals are broccoli, apples, and quinoa.

Another important component of these gut-healing recipes is probiotic-rich foods. Probiotics are beneficial bacteria that can help to restore balance to your gut microbiome and improve digestion. Fermented foods like yogurt, kimchi, and sauerkraut are excellent sources of probiotics and can be easily incorporated into your meals. Adding a serving of probiotic-rich food to your lunch or dinner can help to support a healthy gut and alleviate symptoms of IBS.

In addition to fiber and probiotics, these recipes also focus on incorporating anti-inflammatory ingredients like turmeric, ginger, and garlic. Inflammation in the gut can exacerbate symptoms of IBS, so it's important to include ingredients that can help reduce inflammation and promote healing. By including these anti-inflammatory foods in your meals, you can help to soothe your gut and improve your overall digestive health.

Overall, these gut-healing lunch and dinner recipes are designed to provide you with nourishing and delicious meals that can support your gut health and help alleviate symptoms of IBS. By focusing on fiber, probiotics, and anti-inflammatory ingredients, you can take control of your digestive health and promote healing from the inside out. Give these recipes a try and see how they can benefit your gut and overall well-being.

Snack Ideas for Managing IBS Symptoms

If you suffer from Irritable Bowel Syndrome (IBS), you know how challenging it can be to manage your symptoms on a daily basis. However, one way to help alleviate some of the discomfort associated with IBS is through mindful snacking. By choosing the right foods, you can nourish your gut and help heal your body from the inside out.

When it comes to snacking with IBS, it's important to choose foods that are gentle on the digestive system. Opt for easily digestible options such as rice cakes, plain popcorn, or gluten-free crackers. These snacks are low in FODMAPs, which are carbohydrates that can exacerbate IBS symptoms in some individuals. Additionally, try incorporating small portions of nuts, seeds, or nut butter for a dose of healthy fats and protein.

Another great snack idea for managing IBS symptoms is to include fermented foods in your diet. Fermented foods such as yogurt, kefir, sauerkraut, and kombucha are rich in probiotics, which are beneficial bacteria that can help promote a healthy gut microbiome. These probiotics can help restore balance to your gut and reduce symptoms of IBS such as bloating, gas, and diarrhea.

For those with a sweet tooth, there are plenty of delicious and IBS-friendly snack options to choose from. Try snacking on a piece of dark chocolate, which is lower in sugar and higher in antioxidants compared to milk chocolate. You can also enjoy a small serving of fresh fruit such as berries, bananas, or oranges for a natural and nutritious treat that won't aggravate your IBS symptoms.

In conclusion, incorporating mindful snacking into your daily routine can be a helpful way to manage your IBS symptoms and promote overall gut health. By choosing easily digestible foods, incorporating fermented foods, and enjoying small portions of sweet treats, you can nourish your gut and heal your body from the inside out. Remember to listen to your body and pay attention to how different foods make you feel, as everyone's experience with IBS is unique. With a little experimentation and creativity, you can find snack ideas that work best for you and your individual needs.

Chapter 8: Conclusion

Recap of Key Points

In this subchapter, we will recap some of the key points discussed throughout this book on natural remedies for IBS. Irritable Bowel Syndrome (IBS) is a common digestive disorder that affects the large intestine and can cause symptoms such as bloating, gas, abdominal pain, and changes in bowel habits. One of the key factors in managing IBS is understanding the role of the gut microbiome in maintaining gut health.

The gut microbiome is a complex community of microorganisms that live in the digestive tract and play a crucial role in digestion, immunity, and overall health. Imbalances in the gut microbiome have been linked to various digestive disorders, including IBS. By nourishing your gut with a healthy diet rich in fiber, probiotics, and prebiotics, you can support a diverse and balanced gut microbiome, which may help alleviate symptoms of IBS.

Natural remedies such as herbal supplements, acupuncture, and mindfulness techniques can also be effective in managing IBS symptoms. Herbal remedies like peppermint oil, ginger, and chamomile have been shown to reduce abdominal pain and bloating in individuals with IBS. Acupuncture, a traditional Chinese medicine practice, can help regulate the flow of energy in the body and improve digestive function. Mindfulness techniques such as deep breathing, meditation, and yoga can help reduce stress and anxiety, which are common triggers for IBS symptoms.

It is important to work with a healthcare provider to develop a personalized treatment plan for managing your IBS symptoms. By incorporating natural remedies, nourishing your gut with a healthy diet, and addressing factors that may trigger your symptoms, you can take control of your digestive health and improve your overall well-being. Remember, everyone's experience with IBS is unique, so it may take some trial and error to find the right combination of natural remedies that work best for you. With patience and persistence, you can find relief from IBS and enjoy a healthier gut and body.

Final Thoughts on Nourishing Your Gut and Healing Your Body

In conclusion, it is clear that nourishing your gut and healing your body go hand in hand when it comes to managing IBS. By focusing on incorporating gut-friendly foods such as fiber-rich fruits and vegetables, probiotic-rich fermented foods, and hydrating fluids like water, you can support the health of your gut microbiome and alleviate symptoms of IBS. Additionally, incorporating stress-reducing practices such as meditation, yoga, or deep breathing exercises can also play a significant role in managing IBS symptoms.

It is important to remember that healing your body is a journey, and it may take time to see significant improvements in your IBS symptoms. Patience and consistency in incorporating gut-nourishing practices into your daily routine will ultimately lead to long-lasting results. It is also important to consult with a healthcare provider before making any drastic changes to your diet or lifestyle, especially if you are currently taking medication for IBS.

In addition to nourishing your gut with healthy foods and stress-reducing practices, it is important to explore natural remedies that have been shown to be effective in managing IBS symptoms. Some natural remedies that have shown promise in alleviating IBS symptoms include peppermint oil, ginger, and turmeric. These natural remedies can help reduce inflammation in the gut, alleviate bloating and gas, and improve overall digestion.

Furthermore, it is essential to listen to your body and pay attention to how different foods and lifestyle choices impact your IBS symptoms. Keeping a food diary can be a helpful tool in identifying trigger foods that exacerbate your symptoms. By being mindful of what you eat and how it affects your gut health, you can make informed decisions about what to include in your diet and what to avoid.

In conclusion, nourishing your gut and healing your body is key to managing IBS and improving your overall health and well-being. By incorporating gut-friendly foods, stress-reducing practices, and natural remedies into your daily routine, you can support the health of your gut microbiome and alleviate symptoms of IBS. Remember that healing takes time, so be patient with yourself and seek guidance from a healthcare provider if needed. With dedication and consistency, you can take control of your IBS and live a happier, healthier life.

Resources for Further Information and Support

For those looking for more information and support when it comes to managing IBS and improving gut health, there are a wealth of resources available. Whether you are interested in learning more about the role of the gut microbiome in IBS or exploring natural remedies for symptom relief, there are resources out there to help you on your journey to better health.

One valuable resource for those interested in the gut microbiome and its connection to IBS is the book "The Mind-Gut Connection" by Emeran Mayer. This book delves into the intricate relationship between the brain and the gut, and how disruptions in this connection can lead to digestive issues like IBS. Mayer offers practical advice for improving gut health through diet, lifestyle changes, and stress management techniques.

If you are seeking natural remedies for IBS, the book "Natural Remedies for IBS: Nourish Your Gut, Heal Your Body" is a great resource to explore. This book provides practical tips for incorporating natural remedies like dietary changes, herbal supplements, and mind-body practices into your daily routine to alleviate IBS symptoms and promote overall gut health. The book also includes recipes and meal plans to help you get started on your journey to better digestive health.

In addition to books, there are also online resources available for those seeking more information and support for IBS and gut health. Websites like the International Foundation for Gastrointestinal Disorders (IFFGD) and the American Nutrition Association offer a wealth of information on digestive health, including tips for managing IBS symptoms and improving gut health naturally. These websites also provide access to support groups and forums where you can connect with others who are dealing with similar digestive issues.

Finally, if you are looking for more personalized support in managing your IBS symptoms and improving your gut health, consider reaching out to a qualified healthcare professional. A naturopathic doctor, functional medicine practitioner, or registered dietitian with experience in digestive health can provide personalized guidance and support to help you address the root causes of your digestive issues and develop a comprehensive treatment plan tailored to your unique needs. Remember, you are not alone in your journey to better gut health, and there are resources available to help you every step of the way.